Yoga From Your Chair: Enhance Mobility And Well Being For

Seniors 60 And Up

DISCLAIMER

The information contained in this resource is general in nature and for informative purposes only.

The Author assumes no responsibility whatsoever, under any circumstances, for any actions taken as a result of the information contained herein.

You are required to seek professional help if needed.

Before this document is duplicated or reproduced

in any manner, the publisher's consent must be

gained. Therefore, the contents within can neither

be stored electronically, transferred, nor kept in a

database.

Neither in Part nor full can the document be

copied, scanned, faxed, or retained without

approval from the publisher or creator.

Preface

As we journey through life, our bodies naturally change. The vibrant energy of youth may transition to a slower, more deliberate pace. Yet, within each of us lies an incredible capacity for continued growth and vitality.

This book, "Chair Yoga for Seniors Over 60," is an invitation to embrace that potential. Here, you'll discover the magic of chair yoga, a practice specifically designed to enhance the lives of mature adults.

More than just exercise, chair yoga is a holistic approach to well-being. It weaves together gentle movement, mindful breathing, and relaxation techniques, offering a path to:

- **Improved flexibility and range of motion** to navigate daily activities with ease.
- **Enhanced strength and balance** for increased confidence and a reduced risk of falls.
- **Reduced stress and anxiety** to cultivate inner peace and tranquility.
- **A renewed sense of energy and vitality** to embrace life to the fullest.

No matter your fitness background, chair yoga welcomes you. Whether you've practiced yoga for years or are just starting your exploration of movement, this book provides modifications and guidance to tailor the practice to your unique needs. All you need is a sturdy chair and a willingness to embark on a journey of self-discovery.

Within these pages, you'll find clear instructions, helpful illustrations, and thoughtfully designed routines to guide you on your path. We'll explore the fundamentals of setting up your practice, delve into a variety of chair-adapted poses, and create routines designed to address your specific goals.

This book is more than just a guide; it's a companion on your journey. Let's embark on this adventure together, one gentle movement and mindful breath at a time. As you embrace the practice of chair yoga, you may be surprised by the strength, flexibility, and vitality that awakens within you.

Leo Chambers

Introduction

Welcome to the wonderful world of chair yoga! This gentle and accessible practice offers a multitude of benefits specifically designed to enhance the lives of seniors over 60. Whether you're a seasoned yoga enthusiast or just starting your fitness journey, chair yoga provides a safe and effective way to improve your overall well-being.

Unveiling the Benefits of Chair Yoga:
- **Enhanced Flexibility and Range of Motion:** Gentle movements in the chair help to loosen tight muscles and joints, improving your ability to move with ease and grace.
- **Increased Strength and Balance:** Chair yoga incorporates exercises that target key muscle groups, leading to improved strength, stability, and a reduced risk of falls.
- **Improved Circulation and Energy Levels:** Gentle movements combined with focused breathing promote better blood flow throughout the body, leaving you feeling energized and revitalized.
- **Stress Reduction and Relaxation:** Chair yoga incorporates mindfulness techniques and breathing exercises that help to calm the mind, alleviate stress, and promote feelings of peace and tranquility.

- **Boosted Mood and Well-being**: Regular practice has been shown to improve mood, reduce anxiety and depression symptoms, and enhance overall well-being.
- **Social Connection (Optional Bullet Point)**: Chair yoga classes provide a wonderful opportunity to connect with others in a supportive environment, fostering a sense of community and belonging (consider including this if your book focuses on chair yoga classes).

Getting Started with Ease:
- **No Fancy Equipment Needed:** All you need is a sturdy chair and comfortable clothing to begin your chair yoga practice.
- **Accessible for All Levels:** Whether you're a beginner or have experience with yoga, chair yoga offers modifications to suit your individual needs and abilities.
- **Gentle on Your Body:** The chair provides support and stability, allowing you to enjoy the benefits of yoga without putting strain on your joints.

- **Lifelong Practice:** Chair yoga is a practice you can continue to enjoy well into your golden years.

This book will be your guide on your chair yoga journey. We'll explore the basics of setting up your practice, introduce you to fundamental poses, and create routines designed to address your specific needs. So, grab your chair, take a deep breath, and get ready to embark on a path to greater flexibility, strength, and well-being!

Contents

Acknowledgement

About the Author

Part 1

Embracing Your Chair Yoga Practice

Chapter 1

Cultivating a Sanctuary for Your Chair Yoga Practice

As you embark on your chair yoga adventure, creating a supportive and inviting environment is key to fostering a successful and enjoyable practice. This chapter will guide you through establishing a haven for your well-being, ensuring each session feels enriching and leaves you feeling revitalized.

Crafting a Space for Tranquility:

- **Finding Your Practice Area:** Look for a quiet and clutter-free area in your home where you can move freely without restriction. Ample natural light can be uplifting, while softer lighting can create a more calming atmosphere. Consider using a yoga mat or a comfortable rug to define your practice space.

- **Ensuring Safety and Stability:** Select a sturdy chair with a flat, supportive seat and a backrest that provides moderate support without restricting your movement. Opt for a chair with rubber grips or place a non-slip pad on the bottom of the legs to prevent accidental sliding.
- **Setting the Mood:** Incorporate elements that cultivate a sense of peace and tranquility. Play calming music, light a scented candle with a relaxing aroma, or diffuse essential oils that promote relaxation, such as lavender or chamomile.

Preparing Yourself for Practice:
- **Choosing Comfortable Attire:** Wear loose-fitting clothing that allows for ease of movement. Opt for natural fabrics like cotton or linen that breathe well, especially during warmer weather. Consider wearing socks with good grip to prevent slipping, particularly if you don't use a yoga mat.
- **Embracing Comfort:** Ensure you feel comfortable throughout your practice. Adjust the room temperature to your

preference. Have a bottle of water nearby to stay hydrated, especially during longer sessions.

- **Quieting the Mind**: Take a few moments to settle your mind and establish an inward focus. Begin with a few cycles of deep, cleansing breaths, inhaling through your nose and exhaling slowly through your mouth.

Establishing a Supportive Practice:

- **Listening to Your Body**: Chair yoga is a practice of gentle exploration, not pushing your limits. Pay attention to your body's sensations throughout each pose. If you experience any pain, discomfort, or dizziness, stop the pose and rest. Modifications are always encouraged, so adapt the poses to suit your individual needs and abilities.
- **Respecting Your Pace**: There's no need to rush through your practice. Move slowly and deliberately, focusing on the sensations in your body and the rhythm of your breath. Allow yourself ample time to explore each pose and find stillness within the movement.
- **Celebrating Small Victories**: As with any new endeavor, progress takes time.

Celebrate even the smallest victories, whether it's achieving greater depth in a stretch or holding a pose for a few seconds longer than before.

- **Embracing the Journey:** The practice of chair yoga is a lifelong exploration. Be patient with yourself, and enjoy the process of discovery as you connect with your body and cultivate inner peace.

Additional Tips for Creating a Supportive Practice:

- **Practice Regularly:** Aim for consistent practice, even if it's just for short sessions a few times a week. Regularity is key to reaping the long-term benefits of chair yoga.
- **Find a Yoga Buddy (Optional):** Consider practicing with a friend or joining a chair yoga class. Social interaction can enhance motivation and provide a sense of community.
- **Seek Guidance:** If you have any pre-existing health conditions, consult your doctor before starting a chair yoga practice. A qualified yoga instructor can also provide personalized guidance and modifications.

Remember, your chair yoga practice is a personal journey. By creating a supportive environment and fostering a sense of self-care, you'll establish a foundation for a practice that nourishes your body, mind, and spirit.

Now, let's delve into the fundamentals of chair yoga postures, where we'll explore a variety of gentle movements designed to enhance your flexibility, strength, and overall well-being.

Chapter 2

Building the Bedrock of Your Chair Yoga Practice

Having established a nurturing haven for your practice, it's time to delve into the foundational elements of chair yoga. This chapter will guide you through the cornerstone principles – breathwork, essential postures, and techniques for warming up and cooling down – that will empower you to navigate a safe, effective, and enriching practice.

The Breath of Life: Unveiling the Power of Breathwork

Our breath is a vital link between our body and mind. In chair yoga, mindful breathing, also known as pranayama, plays a crucial role in optimizing the benefits of each pose. By focusing on your breath, you can:

- **Enhance Relaxation:** Controlled, slow breaths activate the parasympathetic nervous system, promoting a sense of calm and well-being.
- **Improve Focus:** Directing your attention to your breath helps to quiet the mind and fosters a state of present-moment awareness.
- **Optimize Movement:** Coordinating your breath with movement allows for smoother transitions and deeper engagement in each pose.

The Art of Pranayama:

Here are two fundamental breathing techniques to integrate into your chair yoga practice:

- **Diaphragmatic Breathing (Belly Breathing):** Sit comfortably in your chair, placing one hand on your chest and the other on your abdomen. As you inhale slowly through your nose, feel your belly expand, pushing your hand outwards. Exhale slowly through pursed lips, allowing your belly to sink inwards as your hand moves back. Practice this technique for several breaths, establishing a steady and effortless rhythm.

- **Dirga Swasham (Three-Part Breath):** Begin in a seated position. Inhale slowly through your nose, feeling your belly expand first, then your chest rise gently. Briefly hold your breath at the peak of your inhalation, then exhale slowly through pursed lips, emptying your belly first, followed by your chest. Repeat this cycle for several breaths, focusing on a smooth and continuous flow of breath.

Mastering the Fundamentals: Essential Chair Yoga Postures

Chair yoga offers a diverse range of postures that can be adapted to suit your individual needs and abilities. Here are some core poses to establish a strong foundation for your practice:

- **Mountain Pose (Tadasana):** Sit tall in your chair with your feet flat on the floor, hip-width apart. Engage your core by gently drawing your belly button towards your spine. Lengthen your spine upwards, maintaining a gentle curve in your lower back. Rest your shoulders back and down, keeping your arms relaxed at your sides. Take a few deep breaths, feeling grounded and centered.

- **Seated Forward Fold (Paschimottanasana):** Sit tall with your feet flat on the floor. Inhale and lengthen your spine. As you exhale, hinge at your hips and gently fold forward, reaching for your shins or the floor (whichever is comfortable) with a flat back. Rest your head on your knees or a block if needed. Hold for a few breaths, focusing on lengthening your spine and releasing tension in your neck and shoulders.
- **Cat-Cow Pose (Marjaryasana-Bitilasana):** Place your hands shoulder-width apart on your thighs and knees directly below your hips. As you inhale, arch your back gently, lifting your head and chest upwards (cow pose). Exhale, rounding your spine towards the ceiling and tucking your chin to your chest (cat pose). Repeat this movement several times, flowing with your breath.

- **Side Bend (Parsvakanasana):** Sit tall in your chair with your feet flat on the floor. Reach your right arm overhead, reaching towards the ceiling. As you exhale, gently bend your torso to the left, reaching your left hand down the side of your chair for support (or rest your hand on your thigh if that's more comfortable). Hold for a few breaths, then repeat on the other side.
- **Eagle Arms (Garudasana):** Sit tall with your feet flat on the floor. Bring your arms out to the sides, then bend your elbows and cross your forearms in front of you, bringing your right arm on top of your left. Wrap your palms together, if possible, or clasp your fingers. Lift your forearms slightly away from your chest and hold for a few breaths. Repeat on the other side.

These are just a few foundational postures to get you started. As you progress in your practice, you can explore a wider range of movements designed to target different muscle groups and enhance your overall well-being.

Warming Up and Cooling Down: Essential Rituals for Safety and Well-being

Just as a car needs to warm up before driving, so does your body before physical activity. A gentle warm-up prepares your muscles for movement improves blood flow, and reduces the risk of injury. Similarly, a cool-down allows your body to gradually return to a resting state and promotes relaxation.

Warming Up:
- **Gentle Neck Rolls:** Slowly roll your head in a circular motion, five times forward and five times backward. Repeat with side-to-side neck rolls.
- **Arm Circles:** Extend your arms out to the sides with palms facing forward. Make small circles with your arms, forward for 10 repetitions, then backward for 10 repetitions. Repeat with palms facing down.
- **Seated Ankle Circles:** Sit tall with your feet flat on the floor. Slowly rotate your ankles clockwise for 10 circles, then counter-clockwise for 10 circles. Repeat on the other side.
- **Seated Twists:** Sit tall with your feet flat on the floor. Inhale and lengthen your spine. Exhale and gently twist your torso to the right, placing your left hand on your right

knee and reaching your right arm back behind you for support (or resting it on the chair back). Hold for a few breaths, then inhale and return to center. Repeat on the other side.

Cooling Down:
- **Seated Forward Fold with Rest:** Sit tall with your feet flat on the floor. Inhale and lengthen your spine. Exhale and gently fold forward, reaching for your shins or the floor (whichever is comfortable) with a flat back. Rest your head on your knees or a block for support. Hold for several breaths, focusing on your breath and releasing any remaining tension.
- **Deep Breathing:** Practice diaphragmatic breathing or three-part breathing for several minutes, allowing your body to gradually come to rest.
- **Progressive Muscle Relaxation:** Tense and release different muscle groups in your body, starting with your toes and working your way up to your head. Hold each tensing for a few seconds, followed by a deep relaxation.

Remember, these are just guidelines. Listen to your body and adjust the duration and intensity of your warm-up and cool-down based on your individual needs.

Building a Foundation for a Fulfilling Practice:

By integrating the principles of breathwork, essential poses, and proper warm-up and cool-down techniques, you've established a strong foundation for your chair yoga journey. As you move forward, remember these key points:

- **Focus on Quality, Not Quantity:** It's not about how many times you can repeat a pose, but rather the quality of your movement and the sensations in your body.
- **Embrace Modifications:** Don't hesitate to modify poses to suit your limitations. Use props like blocks, pillows, or rolled towels for added support.
- **Celebrate Your Progress:** Every step you take on your chair yoga journey is a success. Acknowledge your achievements and enjoy the process of discovery.

With dedication and a playful spirit, chair yoga can become a cherished part of your daily routine, empowering you to cultivate greater flexibility, strength, and a sense of well-being that radiates from within. Now, let's delve into the heart of chair yoga – a variety of invigorating routines designed to address your specific needs and goals.

Part 2
Chair Yoga Poses For Overall Well Being

Chapter 3

Unlocking Suppleness and Freedom of Movement: Improving Flexibility and Range of Motion

Flexibility and range of motion are crucial ingredients for a healthy and functional life. They allow us to navigate daily activities with ease, reduce the risk of falls, and improve our overall posture and balance. Chair yoga offers a gentle and effective way to enhance these qualities, promoting a sense of suppleness and freedom within your body.

Understanding Flexibility and Range of Motion:
- **Flexibility:** Refers to the ability of your muscles to lengthen and stretch, allowing your joints to move through their full range of motion.
- **Range of Motion:** Describes the extent to which a joint can move in a particular direction.

The Benefits of Enhanced Flexibility and Range of Motion:
- **Improved Daily Activities:** Increased flexibility allows you to bend, reach, and twist with greater ease, making everyday tasks like getting dressed, gardening, or picking things up from the floor more manageable.
- **Reduced Risk of Falls:** Tighter muscles can restrict movement and contribute to balance issues. Improved flexibility enhances your

ability to maintain stable positions, reducing the risk of falls.

- **Enhanced Posture and Alignment**: Balanced flexibility throughout your body helps to maintain proper posture and spinal alignment, leading to better comfort and reduced aches and pains.
- **Increased Blood Flow**: Gentle stretching exercises promote circulation, delivering essential nutrients to your muscles and joints, which can aid in healing and reduce stiffness.

A Gentle Approach to Flexibility: Chair Yoga Poses for Enhanced Range of Motion

Chair yoga provides a safe and accessible platform to explore a variety of stretches that target different muscle groups and joints. Here are some key poses to integrate into your practice:

- **Seated Neck Stretches:**
  - **Side Bends:** Sit tall with your feet flat on the floor. Gently bend your head towards your right shoulder, feeling a stretch along the left side of your neck. Hold for a few breaths, then repeat on the other side.

- o **Rotations:** Slowly roll your head in a circular motion, five times forward and five times backward. Focus on keeping your shoulders relaxed throughout the movement.

- **Seated Shoulder Stretches:**
  - o **Eagle Arms:** Sit tall with your feet flat on the floor. Bring your arms out to the sides, then bend your elbows and cross your forearms in front of you, bringing your right arm on top of your left. Wrap your palms together, if possible, or clasp your fingers. Lift your forearms slightly away from your chest and hold for a few breaths. Repeat on the other side.
  - o **Arm Circles:** Extend your arms out to the sides with palms facing forward. Make small circles with your arms, forward for 10 repetitions, then backward for 10 repetitions. Repeat with palms facing down.

- **Seated Torso Twists:**
  - o **Simple Twist:** Sit tall with your feet flat on the floor. Inhale and lengthen

your spine. Exhale and gently twist your torso to the right, placing your left hand on your right knee and reaching your right arm back behind you for support (or resting it on the chair back). Hold for a few breaths, then inhale and return to center. Repeat on the other side.

- **Chair Supported Twist:** Sit sideways on your chair with your feet flat on the floor. Place your right hand on the back of the chair for support and reach your left arm overhead. Gently twist your torso to the right, looking up towards your left hand. Hold for a few breaths, then return to center and repeat on the other side.

- **Seated Leg and Hip Stretches:**
  - **Hamstring Stretch:** Sit tall with your feet flat on the floor. Extend one leg out straight in front of you, keeping the other foot flat on the floor. Flex your pointed toes towards you and gently lean forward from your hips, reaching for your extended foot (or a strap or block if needed). Hold for a

few breaths, then switch legs and repeat.

- ○ **Quad Stretch:** Sit tall with your feet flat on the floor. Lift one foot off the ground and gently pull it towards your chest, placing your hand behind your thigh for support. Hold for a few breaths, then switch legs and repeat.

Remember, these are just a few examples. There are many other chair yoga postures that target different muscle groups. Explore various resources and consult with a qualified yoga instructor for a personalized practice that addresses your specific needs.

Enhancing Your Flexibility Journey

Here are some additional tips to optimize your journey towards greater flexibility and range of motion:

- **Focus on Breath:** Coordinate your breath with your movements. Inhale as you lengthen and exhale as you release, allowing your breath to guide your stretches.
- **Listen to Your Body:** Pain is a signal to stop. Never force a stretch beyond your comfortable range of motion. If you

experience any discomfort, ease up or modify the pose.

- **Hold and Breathe**: Once you reach a comfortable stretch, hold the position for several breaths, allowing your muscles to gently lengthen and release tension.
- **Be Consistent**: Regular practice is key. Aim to incorporate these stretches into your chair yoga routine at least a few times a week for optimal results.
- **Warm Up Before Stretching**: A gentle warm-up prepares your muscles for stretching, making them more receptive and reducing the risk of injury.

Beyond the Poses: Additional Strategies for Flexibility

While chair yoga postures are a valuable tool for improving flexibility, here are some additional strategies to consider:

- **Mind-Body Techniques**: Techniques like progressive muscle relaxation and mindfulness meditation can help you release tension and tightness held within your body.
- **Foam Rolling**: Self-myofascial release techniques using a foam roller can target

specific muscle groups and connective tissues, promoting deeper relaxation and improved flexibility.

- **Staying Hydrated**: Adequate hydration is crucial for maintaining healthy muscle tissue and promoting flexibility. Aim to drink plenty of water throughout the day.

Embrace the Journey of Suppleness:

Remember, improving flexibility is a gradual process. Celebrate even small gains and enjoy the journey of rediscovering freedom of movement in your body. As you continue to practice, you'll likely notice an increased range of motion, improved daily function, and a newfound sense of ease and grace in your movements. The next chapter will delve into another crucial aspect of a well-rounded practice – building strength and balance for enhanced stability and confidence.

Chapter 4

Cultivating Strength and Stability: Building a Foundation for Balance and Confidence

Strength and balance are the cornerstones of a stable and confident body. They allow us to navigate daily activities with ease, reduce the risk of falls, and maintain proper posture and alignment. Chair yoga offers a safe and effective way to build strength in key muscle groups, while simultaneously enhancing our sense of balance and stability.

The Power of Strength and Balance:
- **Strength**: Refers to the ability of your muscles to generate force. Stronger muscles support your joints, improve movement control, and enhance your ability to perform daily activities.
- **Balance**: The ability to maintain your center of gravity over your base of support. Good balance is crucial for preventing falls and maintaining stability during movement.

The Benefits of Building Strength and Balance:
- **Reduced Risk of Falls:** Falls are a major concern for seniors. Enhanced strength and balance reduce the risk of falls and potential injuries.
- **Improved Daily Activities:** Stronger muscles make everyday tasks like carrying groceries, climbing stairs, or getting up from a chair more manageable.

- **Enhanced Posture and Alignment**: Strong core muscles help maintain proper posture and alignment, reducing aches and pains and promoting a sense of well-being.
- **Increased Bone Density**: Regular strength training can help maintain or even increase bone density, which can be beneficial for preventing osteoporosis.

Building Strength with Chair Yoga:

Chair yoga postures, when practiced with intention and proper form, can effectively target various muscle groups throughout your body. Here are some key poses to integrate into your practice for strength development:

- **Upper Body Strengthening Poses:**
    - **Chair Push-ups**: Sit on the edge of your chair with your hands shoulder-width apart on the armrests. Straighten your legs and press down through your palms, as if doing a push-up from a seated position. Lower yourself back down slowly with control. Modify by keeping your knees bent if needed.
    - **Bicep Curls with Weights (Optional)**: Sit tall in your chair with your feet flat on the floor. Hold light weights (water

bottles can be used) in each hand. Curl your weights up towards your shoulders, squeezing your biceps muscles. Slowly lower the weights back down with control.

- **Core Strengthening Poses:**
  - ○ **Seated Abdominal Crunches:** Sit tall in your chair with your feet flat on the floor. Lean back slightly, engaging your core muscles. Lift your shoulders off the chair slightly, keeping your lower back pressed against the backrest. Slowly lower yourself back down with control. Modify by keeping your hands behind your head for support if needed.
  - ○ **Seated Side Bends with Weights (Optional):** Sit tall in your chair with your feet flat on the floor. Hold a light weight (water bottle can be used) in your right hand. Lean to your left side, reaching your right arm overhead as you engage your obliques. Hold for a few breaths, then return to center and repeat on the other side.

- **Lower Body Strengthening Poses:**
  - **Chair Squats:** Stand up from your chair, holding onto the backrest for support if needed. Slowly lower yourself back down as if sitting in a chair, keeping your core engaged and your knees tracking over your toes. Push back up to standing with control. Modify by performing smaller squats or sitting down only partially if needed.
  - **Calf Raises:** Stand behind your chair with your hands resting on the backrest for support. Rise up onto your toes, feeling the work in your calves. Slowly lower yourself back down with control. Repeat for several repetitions.

Remember, these are just a few examples. There are many other chair yoga postures that target different muscle groups. Explore various resources and consult with a qualified yoga instructor for a personalized practice that addresses your specific needs and abilities

.

Enhancing Your Strength-Building Journey:

Here are some additional tips to maximize your strength-building journey with chair yoga:

- **Focus on Form**: Proper form is crucial for maximizing benefits and preventing injury. Pay attention to body alignment during each pose and don't hesitate to modify if needed.
- **Start Light and Gradually Increase Intensity**: Begin with lighter weights or bodyweight exercises and gradually increase the intensity as your strength improves.
- **Focus on Control**: Move slowly and with control throughout each exercise. Emphasis on controlled movements is more effective for building strength than jerky or rushed motions.
- **Consistency is Key**: Regular practice is essential for building and maintaining strength. Aim to incorporate these strengthening exercises into your chair yoga routine at least a few times a week.

Building Balance with Confidence

Chair yoga offers a unique platform to explore balance poses in a safe and controlled environment with the support of the chair. Here are some key poses to integrate into your practice for enhanced balance:

- **Single-Leg Standing Poses:**

- **Tree Pose (Vrksasana) with Chair Support:** Stand next to your chair with one hand resting on the backrest for support. Slowly lift one foot off the ground and bring your knee towards your chest. Balance on your standing leg and gently place your lifted foot on your inner calf, ankle, or shin (whichever is comfortable). Hold for a few breaths, then switch legs and repeat.
  - **Heel-Toe Stand with Chair Support:** Stand next to your chair with one hand resting on the backrest for support. Lift one heel off the ground and bring it to touch the toes of your standing foot. Maintain a tall posture and hold for a few breaths. Switch legs and repeat.

- **Seated Balancing Poses:**
  - **Eagle Arms with Eyes Closed (Optional):** Sit tall with your feet flat on the floor. Bring your arms out to the sides, then bend your elbows and cross your forearms in front of you, bringing your right arm on top of your left.

Wrap your palms together, if possible, or clasp your fingers. Lift your forearms slightly away from your chest and close your eyes for a few breaths, focusing on maintaining your balance. Repeat on the other side.

- **Seated Figure-Four Stretch with Twist:** Sit tall in your chair with your feet flat on the floor. Cross your right ankle over your left thigh, just above your knee. Lean slightly forward and reach your right arm towards your left foot (or a block or strap if needed) for support. Hold for a few breaths, then switch legs and repeat on the other side.

- **Standing Balancing Poses with Chair Support (Optional):** As you progress in your practice and feel confident, you can explore standing balancing poses with the chair nearby for support if needed. Examples include Warrior I (Virabhadrasana I) or Mountain Pose (Tadasana) on one leg.

Remember, these are just a few examples. There are many other chair yoga postures that challenge your balance in a safe and controlled manner. Explore various resources and consult with a qualified yoga instructor for a personalized practice that addresses your specific needs and comfort level.

Enhancing Your Balance Journey:

Here are some additional tips to optimize your journey towards improved balance:

- **Focus on Your Breath:** Coordinate your breath with your movements. Inhale as you initiate the pose and exhale as you hold it, allowing your breath to anchor you and enhance your focus.
- **Start with Eyes Open and Progress to Eyes Closed:** Initially, practice balancing poses with your eyes open to establish a sense of stability. As you gain confidence, gradually progress to closing your eyes for a greater challenge to your proprioception (your body's awareness of its position in space).
- **Challenge Yourself Gradually:** Don't be afraid to step outside your comfort zone, but do so gradually. As your balance improves, try more challenging variations of poses or standing for longer durations.

- **Practice Makes Progress**: Regular practice is essential for improving balance. Aim to incorporate these balancing exercises into your chair yoga routine at least a few times a week.

Building Strength and Balance for a Life in Motion:

By incorporating strength and balance exercises into your chair yoga practice, you're laying the foundation for a more confident and independent life. Enhanced strength allows you to navigate daily activities with ease, while improved balance reduces the risk of falls and fosters a sense of security. Remember, progress takes time, so celebrate your achievements, big and small, and enjoy the journey of building a strong and stable body that supports you in all aspects of life.

The next chapter will delve into the realm of relaxation and mindfulness, exploring techniques that promote inner peace and well-being, further enriching your chair yoga practice.

Chapter 5

Cultivating Inner Peace: Promoting Relaxation and Mindfulness in Chair Yoga

The world around us can be a whirlwind of activity and stress. Chair yoga offers a sanctuary to cultivate relaxation and mindfulness, promoting a sense of inner peace that transcends the physical postures. By integrating these practices into your routine, you'll not only enhance the benefits of your movements but also cultivate a sense of well-being that resonates throughout your day.

The Power of Relaxation and Mindfulness:
- **Relaxation**: The ability to release physical and mental tension, promoting a sense of calmness and tranquility.
- **Mindfulness**: The practice of focusing your attention on the present moment, without judgment, fostering a sense of awareness and acceptance.

The Benefits of Relaxation and Mindfulness:
- **Reduced Stress and Anxiety:** Chronic stress can wreak havoc on your physical and mental health. Relaxation techniques and mindfulness practices can help to quiet the mind, reduce stress hormones, and promote a sense of calm.
- **Improved Sleep Quality:** Stress and a busy mind can often lead to restless nights. Relaxation techniques can help to prepare your body and mind for sleep, promoting deeper and more restorative rest.
- **Enhanced Focus and Concentration:** Mindfulness practices train your attention to stay present in the moment, reducing distractions and improving your ability to focus on the task at hand.
- **Increased Self-Awareness:** By focusing your attention inwards, mindfulness practices can enhance your awareness of your thoughts, emotions, and bodily sensations, empowering you to respond to life's challenges with greater clarity and equanimity.

Integrating Relaxation and Mindfulness into Your Chair Yoga Practice:

Here are some techniques to incorporate relaxation and mindfulness into your chair yoga routine:

- **Mindful Breathing:** Breathwork, also known as pranayama, is the cornerstone of mindful movement in chair yoga. Focus on slow, deep, and diaphragmatic breathing throughout your practice. Feel your belly expand with each inhalation and gently contract with each exhalation. Let your breath be a soothing anchor that guides your movements and quiets your mind.

- **Body Scan Meditation:** While seated comfortably in your chair, close your eyes (if comfortable) or soften your gaze. Begin by bringing your awareness to your toes and feet. Notice any sensations present, without judgment. Gradually scan your body upwards, paying attention to each muscle group and bodily region. Observe any tightness, tension, or relaxation. Continue this process until you've scanned your entire body.

- **Guided Imagery:** Guided imagery involves using visualizations to create a sense of relaxation and peace. Find a guided imagery recording that resonates with you, or simply close your eyes and visualize a calming scene, such as a peaceful beach or a serene forest. Engage your senses in the visualization, noticing the sights, sounds, smells, and textures of your imaginary environment. Allow yourself to fully immerse yourself in the experience, promoting a sense of relaxation and inner peace.

- **Movement with Awareness:** Approach each chair yoga pose with a sense of mindful awareness. Focus on the sensations in your body as you move. Notice the alignment of your joints, the engagement of your muscles, and the breath flowing through your body. Move slowly and deliberately, savoring each movement and being fully present in the here and now.

Remember, these are just a few techniques. There are many other relaxation and mindfulness practices you can explore to further enrich your chair yoga experience. Consult with a qualified yoga instructor or therapist for personalized guidance.

Enhancing Your Relaxation and Mindfulness Journey:

Here are some additional tips to optimize your journey towards inner peace:

- **Create a Relaxing Environment:** Dim the lights, light some soothing candles, or diffuse calming essential oils like lavender or chamomile to create a tranquil atmosphere for your practice.
- **Practice Regularly:** Like any skill, relaxation and mindfulness require consistent practice to reap the long-term benefits. Aim to integrate these techniques into your chair yoga routine at least a few times a week.
- **Be Patient:** Don't get discouraged if your mind wanders during your practice. Gently redirect your attention back to the present moment without judgment. With consistent practice, you'll find it easier to cultivate a sense of calm and focus.
- **Extend the Benefits Beyond Your Practice:** The benefits of relaxation and mindfulness aren't limited to your yoga mat. Try incorporating these techniques throughout your day to manage stress, improve focus, and cultivate a sense of inner peace in all aspects of your life.

Cultivating a Sanctuary Within:
By integrating relaxation and mindfulness practices into your chair yoga routine, you're creating a sanctuary within yourself. This inner sanctuary will serve as a refuge from the daily stresses of life, promoting a sense of peace, well-being, and a newfound appreciation for the present moment. As you embark on this journey of self-discovery, remember to embrace the process. There will be days when achieving a state of perfect relaxation seems elusive. That's perfectly alright. The key is to keep practicing, to cultivate self-compassion, and to celebrate even the smallest moments of inner peace.

The next chapter will delve into the concept of creating a sustainable chair yoga practice, offering tips and strategies to integrate this practice seamlessly into your life and empower you to reap the long-term benefits of chair yoga for years to come.

Part 3
Putting All Together

Chapter 6

Building a Sustainable Practice: Sample Chair Yoga Routines and Tips for Long-Term Success

Having explored the foundational elements of chair yoga and their associated benefits, it's time to translate theory into practice. This chapter will provide you with a variety of sample chair yoga routines designed to target different needs and goals. Additionally, we'll delve into practical tips for establishing a sustainable practice, empowering you to integrate chair yoga seamlessly into your daily life and experience its transformative power for years to come.

Sample Chair Yoga Routines:
Here are a few sample chair yoga routines to get you started. Remember, these are just a starting point. Feel free to modify the postures, adjust the duration, and create your own routines based on your individual needs and preferences.

Gentle Morning Routine (15-20 minutes):
- **Warm-Up (5 minutes):**
    - **Neck Rolls:** Slowly roll your head in a circular motion, five times forward and five times backward. Repeat with side-to-side neck rolls.
    - **Arm Circles:** Extend your arms out to the sides with palms facing forward. Make small circles with your arms,

forward for 10 repetitions, then backward for 10 repetitions. Repeat with palms facing down.

- **Seated Stretches (5 minutes):**
    - **Seated Forward Fold (Paschimottanasana):** Sit tall with your feet flat on the floor. Inhale and lengthen your spine. As you exhale, gently fold forward, reaching for your shins or the floor (whichever is comfortable) with a flat back. Rest your head on your knees or a block for support. Hold for a few breaths.
    - **Seated Cat-Cow Pose (Marjaryasana-Bitilasana):** Place your hands shoulder-width apart on your thighs and knees directly below your hips. As you inhale, arch your back gently, lifting your head and chest upwards (cow pose). Exhale, rounding your spine towards the ceiling and tucking your chin to your chest (cat pose). Repeat this movement several times.
    - **Seated Side Bends (Parsvakanasana):** Sit tall with your feet flat on the floor. Reach your right arm overhead, reaching towards the ceiling. As you

exhale, gently bend your torso to the left, placing your left hand on your chair for support (or rest your hand on your thigh if that's more comfortable). Hold for a few breaths, then repeat on the other side.

- **Balance Poses (5 minutes):**
    - **Single-Leg Stand with Chair Support (optional):** Stand next to your chair with one hand resting on the backrest for support. Slowly lift one foot off the ground and bring your knee towards your chest. Balance on your standing leg for a few breaths, then switch legs and repeat.

- **Cool-Down (5 minutes):**
    - **Seated Forward Fold with Rest:** Sit tall with your feet flat on the floor. Inhale and lengthen your spine. Exhale and gently fold forward, reaching for your shins or the floor (whichever is comfortable) with a flat back. Rest your head on your knees or a block for support. Hold for several breaths.

- o **Deep Breathing:** Practice diaphragmatic breathing or three-part breathing for several minutes, allowing your body to gradually come to rest.

Energizing Afternoon Routine (20-25 minutes):
- **Warm-Up (5 minutes):**
  - o Same as Gentle Morning Routine.
- **Strengthening Poses (10 minutes):**
  - o **Chair Push-ups:** Sit on the edge of your chair with your hands shoulder-width apart on the armrests. Straighten your legs and press down through your palms, as if doing a push-up from a seated position. Lower yourself back down slowly with control. Modify by keeping your knees bent if needed.
  - o **Seated Abdominal Crunches:** Sit tall in your chair with your feet flat on the floor. Lean back slightly, engaging your core muscles. Lift your shoulders off the chair slightly, keeping your lower back pressed against the backrest. Slowly lower yourself back down with control. Modify by keeping your hands

behind your head for support if needed.
  - **Chair Squats**: Stand up from your chair, holding onto the backrest for support if needed. Slowly lower yourself back down as if sitting in a chair, keeping your core engaged and your knees tracking over your toes. Push back up to standing with control. Modify by performing smaller squats or sitting down only partially if needed.

- **Balance Poses with Challenge (5 minutes):**
  - **Tree Pose (Vrksasana) with Limited Chair Support:** Stand next to your chair with your hand lightly resting on the backrest for minimal support. Slowly lift one foot off the ground and bring your knee towards your chest. Balance on your standing leg and gently place your lifted foot on your inner calf, ankle, or shin (whichever is comfortable). Hold for a few breaths, then switch legs and repeat.

- **Cool-Down (5 minutes):**
  - Same as Gentle Morning Routine.

Restorative Evening Routine (15-20 minutes):

- **Warm-Up (5 minutes):**
  - Gentle Neck Rolls and Arm Circles (optional): As described in the Gentle Morning Routine.
- **Seated Stretches with Props (10 minutes):**
  - **Seated Forward Fold with Strap or Block:** Sit tall with your feet flat on the floor. Loop a yoga strap or place a block a few feet in front of you. Inhale and lengthen your spine. Exhale and gently fold forward, reaching for the strap or block with a flat back. Rest your head on your arms or a folded blanket for support. Hold for several breaths.
  - **Supported Supine Twist (Supta Matsyendrasana) with Bolster (optional):** Lie on your back on the floor with your knees bent and feet flat on the floor. Place a bolster or rolled-up blanket next to you. Gently extend your right leg out straight and bring your left knee across your body, resting your left foot on the floor beside your right hip. Turn your head to gaze to the

right and extend your right arm out to the side with your palm facing down. Hold for a few breaths, then switch sides.

- **Relaxation Techniques (5 minutes):**
  - ○ **Guided Imagery:** Close your eyes (if comfortable) and visualize a calming scene, such as a peaceful beach or a serene forest. Engage your senses in the visualization, noticing the sights, sounds, smells, and textures of your imaginary environment. Allow yourself to fully immerse yourself in the experience, promoting a sense of relaxation and inner peace.
  - ○ **Body Scan Meditation:** While seated comfortably in your chair, close your eyes (if comfortable) or soften your gaze. Begin by bringing your awareness to your toes and feet. Notice any sensations present, without judgment. Gradually scan your body upwards, paying attention to each muscle group and bodily region. Observe any tightness, tension, or relaxation.

Continue this process until you've scanned your entire body.

Remember, these are just a few examples. There are countless variations and modifications you can explore to create chair yoga routines that cater to your specific needs and preferences.

Building a Sustainable Chair Yoga Practice:

Here are some practical tips to establish a sustainable chair yoga practice and integrate it seamlessly into your daily life:

- **Find a Time that Works for You**: Whether it's first thing in the morning, during your lunch break, or before bed, choose a time that fits comfortably into your schedule. Consistency is key, so aim to practice at least a few times a week.
- **Start Small and Gradually Increase**: Begin with shorter routines (10-15 minutes) and gradually increase the duration as your fitness and comfort level improve.
- **Listen to Your Body**: Pay attention to your body's signals. Don't push yourself beyond your limits. If you experience any pain, modify the pose or take a break.

- **Create a Dedicated Space (Optional):** While not essential, having a dedicated space for your chair yoga practice can help establish a sense of routine and focus. Choose a quiet area with enough space to move comfortably.
- **Invest in a Comfortable Chair:** A sturdy chair with good back support is ideal for your practice.
- **Find a Yoga Buddy (Optional):** Practicing with a friend or family member can add a social element and increase motivation.
- **Track Your Progress:** Keeping a simple journal to track your progress can be a great source of motivation. Note down the routines you practice, any improvements you notice, and how you're feeling overall.
- **Embrace the Journey:** Chair yoga is a journey, not a destination. There will be days when you feel more motivated than others. The key is to be kind to yourself, celebrate your progress, and enjoy the process of cultivating a healthy and mindful practice.

Conclusion:

Chair yoga offers a transformative and accessible approach to improving your overall well-being. By incorporating the principles outlined in this guide, you can create a sustainable practice that empowers you to cultivate strength, flexibility, balance, relaxation, and mindfulness. With dedication and a playful spirit, chair yoga can become a cherished ritual that enhances your life on and off the chair.

Remember, the most important aspect of your practice is to find joy in the movement and to embrace the journey of self-discovery that unfolds with each breath and each pose. Namaste!

Additional Resources:

This chapter has provided a foundation for exploring the world of chair yoga. To further enrich your practice, consider these resources:

- **Online Chair Yoga Classes:** Numerous online platforms offer chair yoga classes for all levels. Explore different instructors and styles to find what resonates with you.
- **Yoga DVDs or Streaming Services:** There are a variety of chair yoga DVDs and streaming services available that offer guided routines and instructional videos.
- **Books on Chair Yoga:** Several books delve deeper into the practice of chair yoga,

offering detailed instructions, modifications, and variations for different needs.

- **Certified Chair Yoga Instructor**: Consider working with a certified chair yoga instructor who can create a personalized practice plan and provide guidance on proper form and alignment.

Remember, the world of chair yoga is vast and ever-evolving. Embrace the opportunity to explore, experiment, and discover the routines and techniques that bring you the greatest benefit and joy. As you embark on this transformative journey, may you find strength, flexibility, balance, and a sense of inner peace that permeates every aspect of your life.

Chapter 7

Cultivating Consistency and Confidence: Staying Motivated and Safe in Your Chair Yoga Practice

Maintaining enthusiasm and prioritizing safety are fundamental aspects of establishing a long-term chair yoga practice. This chapter will equip you with strategies to keep your practice engaging and fulfilling while minimizing the risk of injury.

Maintaining Motivation on Your Chair Yoga Journey:

Motivation is the spark that ignites your practice and keeps you coming back for more. Here are some tips to cultivate consistent motivation:

- **Set SMART Goals:** **S**pecific, **M**easurable, **A**ttainable, **R**elevant, and **T**ime-bound goals provide direction and a sense of accomplishment. For example, you might set a goal to practice chair yoga for 15 minutes, three times a week for the next month.
- **Focus on the Benefits:** Remind yourself of the positive changes chair yoga brings to your life. Jot down how you feel after practicing, noting improvements in flexibility, strength, or mood. Refer back to these notes when motivation wanes.
- **Find Inspiration:** Immerse yourself in the world of chair yoga. Explore online chair yoga communities, watch inspirational videos, or

read success stories of others who have benefited from this practice.

- **Celebrate Milestones**: Acknowledge and celebrate your achievements, big and small. Reaching a new personal best in holding a pose or simply completing a full routine are all reasons to feel proud.
- **Make it Fun**: Choose routines you enjoy and explore different variations to keep things interesting. Play upbeat music during your practice or add a touch of lightheartedness with playful poses.
- **Practice with a Friend (Optional)**: Having a yoga buddy can add a social element and boost accountability. Find a friend or family member to practice with, or join an online chair yoga class for a sense of community.
- **Track Your Progress**: Keeping a simple journal to track your practice can be a powerful motivator. Note down the routines you perform, any improvements you observe, and how you're feeling overall. Reviewing your progress can highlight your dedication and inspire you to continue.

Prioritizing Safety in Your Chair Yoga Practice:

Safety is paramount in chair yoga, especially for those who are new to exercise or have any physical limitations. Here are some key safety principles to follow:

- **Listen to Your Body**: Your body is your wisest guide. Pay close attention to any sensations you experience during your practice. If you feel any pain, stop the pose and rest. Don't push yourself beyond your comfortable limits.
- **Start Slow and Gradually Increase Intensity**: Begin with shorter, beginner-friendly routines and gradually increase the duration and difficulty as your strength and flexibility improve.
- **Choose a Sturdy Chair**: Select a stable chair with a good back support for your practice. Avoid chairs with wheels or swivel bases, as these can pose a safety risk.
- **Warm Up Before You Begin**: Prepare your body for movement with gentle stretches and light cardio exercises. A warm-up helps to increase blood flow, improve flexibility, and reduce the risk of injury.
- **Maintain Proper Form**: Focus on proper alignment during each pose. If you're unsure about a specific movement, don't hesitate to

modify it or skip it altogether. Consider working with a certified chair yoga instructor to learn proper form and technique.

- **Hydrate:** Drink plenty of water before, during, and after your practice. Proper hydration is crucial for optimal performance and injury prevention.
- **Be Mindful of Limitations:** If you have any pre-existing health conditions, consult with your doctor before starting a chair yoga practice. They can advise you on any modifications or limitations you may need to follow.
- **Don't Be Afraid to Modify:** Chair yoga is adaptable to various needs and abilities. Don't be afraid to modify poses to suit your comfort level. There are always alternative ways to experience the benefits of the pose.

Remember, these are just a starting point. As you continue your chair yoga journey, you'll develop a deeper understanding of your body and its needs. Listen to your intuition, prioritize safety, and don't hesitate to seek guidance from a qualified instructor if needed.

The Journey Continues:
Chair yoga is a lifelong exploration, offering a gateway to enhanced physical and mental well-being. By prioritizing motivation and safety, you can cultivate a sustainable practice that empowers you to move with greater ease, find inner peace, and experience the transformative power of chair yoga. Embrace the journey, celebrate your progress, and enjoy the countless benefits this practice has to offer.

Additional Resources:
This chapter has provided a roadmap for staying motivated and safe in your chair yoga practice. To further enhance your experience, consider these resources:

- **Online Chair Yoga Communities:** Several online platforms offer forums and groups dedicated to chair yoga. These communities provide a space to connect with others who share your passion, ask questions, and offer support and encouragement.
- **Motivational Podcasts:** Listen to podcasts that focus on health, wellness, and maintaining a positive mindset. These inspirational talks can provide a much-needed

boost of motivation when you're feeling discouraged.

- **Chair Yoga Apps:** There are a variety of chair yoga apps available that offer guided routines, instructional videos, and progress tracking tools. Explore different apps to find one that suits your needs and preferences.
- **Workshops and Retreats (Optional):** Consider attending chair yoga workshops or retreats for an immersive experience. These events offer a chance to learn from experienced instructors, connect with a like-minded community, and deepen your practice in a supportive environment.

By incorporating these resources and strategies, you can transform your chair yoga practice into a vibrant and sustainable source of well-being, motivation, and self-discovery. As you embark on this transformative journey, remember to embrace the present moment, celebrate your progress, and find joy in the movement. Namaste!

Conclusion

Chair yoga offers a unique and accessible path to cultivating a healthier and happier life. This comprehensive guide has equipped you with the knowledge and tools to embark on this transformative journey. Remember, chair yoga is a practice, not a destination. Be patient with yourself, celebrate your achievements, and embrace the joy of movement.

As you step forward on your chair yoga adventure, keep these key takeaways in mind:
- **Strength and balance are the cornerstones of a stable and confident body.** Chair yoga postures effectively target various muscle groups, enhancing your strength and promoting a sense of balance.
- **Relaxation and mindfulness are essential for inner peace.** Integrate breathing

techniques and meditation practices into your routine to cultivate a sense of calm and well-being.

- **Building a sustainable practice is key to long-term benefits.** Find a time that works for you, start slow and gradually increase intensity, and prioritize safety by listening to your body and practicing proper form.
- **Stay motivated and celebrate your progress.** Set achievable goals, track your progress, and find inspiration in the countless benefits chair yoga offers.

Embrace the opportunity to explore, experiment, and discover the routines and techniques that bring you the greatest joy and fulfillment. May your chair yoga practice become a cherished ritual that empowers you to navigate life with greater strength, flexibility, and a sense of inner peace. Namaste!

Appendix

Glossary of Yoga Terms

Asana (AH-sah-nah): Physical posture or pose.

Bandha (BAN-dah): Internal energetic lock engaged by specific muscle contractions.

Chakra (CHAH-kra): Energy center in the body believed to be associated with specific physiological and psychological functions. Common chakras include the root chakra, sacral chakra, solar plexus chakra, heart chakra, throat chakra, third eye chakra, and crown chakra.

Drishti (DRISH-tee): Focal point for the gaze during yoga practice.

Hatha Yoga (HA-tha): The branch of yoga focused on physical postures (asanas) and breathing exercises (pranayama).

Mantra (MAN-tra): Sacred sound, word, or phrase used in meditation for focus and spiritual connection.

Mudra (MOO-dra): Symbolic hand gesture used in yoga practice.

Namaste (NAH-mah-stay): Traditional Sanskrit greeting that translates to "the divine in me bows to the divine in you."

Pranayama (prah-nah-YAH-mah): Yogic breathing exercises that control the breath for physical and mental benefits.

Samarasa (sah-MAH-rah-sah): State of equanimity or evenness of mind.

Savasana (shah-VAH-sah-nah): Corpse pose; a relaxation pose typically practiced at the end of a yoga session.

Sanskrit: Ancient Indo-European language considered the sacred language of Hinduism and yoga.

Shanti (SHAHN-tee): Peace.

Tadasana (tah-DAH-sah-nah): Mountain pose; a basic standing pose with the feet together and arms at the sides.

Vinyasa (vi-NYAH-sah): Flow or connection; refers to the practice of linking breath with movement in a smooth, flowing sequence.

Yin Yoga: A style of yoga that focuses on holding passive floor postures for extended periods of time to target connective tissues and improve flexibility.

Yogi/Yogini (YOH-ghee/YOH-gi-nee):
Practitioner of yoga.

Please note: This is not an exhaustive list of yoga terms. There are many other terms and concepts used in yoga practice.

Acknowledgement

I wish to thank Almighty God for the inspiration to undertake this project and contribute to the society positively.

About the Author

Leo Chambers is a creative writer and Digital Content Creator.